Top 5 Ways
To Take Your Sex Life
From Great…
To WOW!!

~Misti McCloud

Top 5 Ways To Take Your Sex Life From Great…To WOW! By Misti McCloud

Books may be purchased in quantity and/or special sales by contacting the publisher, Great2Wow Press, by email at great2wow@gmail.com.

Published by: Great2Wow Press, Asheville, NC
Cover Design by: Steven Chrystal, Misti McCloud
Editing by: Misti McCloud
Author's Bio Photo: Marilyn O'Connell

ISBN-13: 978-1502447333
10 9 8 7 6 5 4 3 2 1

Table of Contents

Dearest Reader,

Inside these pages lies essential information you need to know to **empower yourself** by improving your sex life.

You may have a perfectly good sex life. In fact, you may even think it's great. But let's face it – no matter how awesome your sex life is now, wouldn't you love to enhance it?

This book is an *indispensible* guide to improving your sex life and, even if it's great, take it to WOW!

I wrote this book because your well-being depends, among other things, on making choices about your own body and taking control of your own pleasure.

Assuming ownership of your own sexuality is one of the most important ways you can be empowered.

Whether you are heterosexual or homosexual, in a committed relationship or single, I want to help you break through your existing constraints and restrictions, and radically increase the pleasures and possibilities of your own sexuality.

Each chapter provides honest, no-nonsense guidance, as well as valuable resources and tips; all geared towards helping you improve the quality of your sexual experiences and increase the level of "juiciness" in your life.

With your intention, passion, and willingness to love yourself, you **can** reach a new level of sensual awareness and sexual happiness. And, even if your sex life is already great (*and I hope it is*), this book will help you take it to WOW.

Here's to your empowerment,

Misti McCloud

Now then - On to Chapter One!

1. Be Juicy
(and become irresistible)

Smiling regularly.

Carrying yourself with pride.

Comfortably saying hello to (and chatting with) strangers.

Do you do any of these things on a regular basis? If so, it's possible you're already a juicy woman, or at least on your way to becoming one.

Even if you're already juicy, you can become *completely irresistible* with just a few small tweaks.

However, even if you don't consider yourself a juicy woman, thanks to this book you **can easily become one**!

First, you may be wondering just what the heck I mean when I refer to a woman as being "juicy?"

Good question!

A juicy woman has a spring in her step and liveliness about her. She's that woman people want to talk with, be around, and who exudes a sense of excitement. A juicy woman usually has a passion and curiosity for the world around her.

Above all, juicy women everywhere share three core characteristics:

- ✓ A ready smile and a direct gaze
- ✓ A light-hearted approach to life and its challenges
- ✓ A persistently positive and self-confident demeanor

At first glance, these may seem like relatively straightforward qualities. In fact, you may think you're pretty well set in these areas. If so, feel free to skip to the next chapter.

If, however, you want to increase your juiciness level and become *irresistible* (or even if you're just curious), read on!

First, it's helpful to address the "why" of being juicy. If you (like me) were one of those kids in school who bugged teachers by asking "why" all the time, you're going to love this!

Here's the brass tacks question: *"Why is being juicy important?"*

My rather blunt, tongue-in-cheek answer would be to simply tell you that it's the best alternative to being boring. And nobody wants to be boring, let alone have sex with a boring person. Right?

***WARNING!!! If you *want* to be boring, do **not** follow the advice in this book!

You're still here? Great! Let's jump right in, and begin with the ready smile and direct gaze.

You'd think this would be the easy part, right? Instead, this bit can be quite challenging, but I have some *key insights* that will help you.

For instance, start with your smile.

They say a smile is the light in the window of your face that tells people you're at home. Trust me - you *want* people to know you're at home!

With the right smile, your light will burn so brightly people won't be able to help themselves – they'll notice you. And, like the proverbial moth to a flame, they'll be drawn to you.

I'm not saying you need to always smile so hard your face hurts and you can never have any other expression. That's just ridiculous (and pretty creepy). Instead, focus on the *kind* of smile you put on your face, and then pay attention to *how often* you wear it.

Are you wondering what I mean when I refer to the *kind* of smile you're wearing? That's a good question!

Have you ever met someone whose mouth was smiling, but their smile didn't quite reach their eyes? Or have you had someone smile at you in a way you just *knew* wasn't honest or genuine? Maybe it was even condescending?

Clearly, those are **not** the smiles worn by juicy women. Don't even put those types of fake smiles in your handbag in the morning – just leave them at home.

Now – think about the way you might smile at an adorable puppy/kitten/favorite baby animal. If you don't automatically know what that smile feels like on your face, borrow a friend's puppy/kitten/favorite baby animal, have a mirror present, and watch your expression - so you can get to know your face and how it looks & feels when you're wearing a *genuine* smile.

That's the smile I'm talking about! That smile – right there!

After you know what that smile looks/feels like, practice putting it on your face; *even when you don't have a puppy/kitten/favorite baby animal around.* Yes, you might feel silly – but who cares? Do it when nobody is looking!

Once you've got it, make sure you practice that smile until you can put it on easily - even in the middle of a crowded subway train full of boring people – and without thinking about it. Make that smile second nature; make it your new best friend.

Did you know a smile can be seen from twice the distance of other expressions?

This means people you may not even see will be able to notice you when you're smiling. Also, smiles are contagious (kind of like yawns, only better).

When people see you smiling, they are much *more* likely to smile back at you. How cool is that?

Make sure you take opportunities to walk around the world with that smile at the ready (not necessarily plastered on your face 100% of the time, though). Pay attention to what happens when you wear your smile. I bet you'll see a noticeable difference in how people respond to you.

Trust me – this will have a domino effect in taking your daily interactions from great...to wow!

You may be thinking that smiling at people is great and everything, but how does smiling help your sex life? After all, isn't that what this book is about?

You're right – this *is* about taking your sex life from great to wow, but as with anything else, you need a good foundation upon which to build.

Take a moment and think about it. Who are the people you find most attractive? If presented with two potential partners – one who doesn't smile (and possibly even frowns a lot) or one who has that ready, open smile - who would *you* rather have sex with? I don't know about you, but unless it's someone like Billy Idol (who always has that sexy sneer going on), I will always choose the person who smiles!

The same goes for the majority of people. So, as it turns out, that most basic of things – the ready and open smile – *automatically makes you increasingly attractive to more people.* I won't do the math on that (I'm a writer), but I can pretty much guarantee you will exponentially increase your number of potential partners, **and** expand your chances for some really great sex that leaves you saying "wow!"

Now then, what about that direct gaze?

If you're like many people, meeting someone's gaze can be quite uncomfortable if you're not used to it. Believe it or not, you don't have to have a staring contest with everyone you meet (that's annoying). The mere act of meeting their gaze directly for a brief second will get the message across that you're paying attention to them. If you hold their gaze for a full two or three seconds, you can clearly communicate that you're not only interested in what they have to say, but in who they are as a person.

Combining an open and direct gaze with the smile you've now mastered will definitely take your connections from great…to wow!

Important note: When you're with your partner, a lover, or someone with whom you want to be intimate, feel free to have fun with it. For example, waggling your eyebrows a bit can be playfully suggestive and help get things going. If you're feeling really bold, let your gaze move steadily and intentionally from their eyes over their body. Don't be lecherous about it, though – there are ways to be tasteful but still get your sexy message across.

Fair warning: you may find this has an enormously empowering side effect!

Regardless of your sexual orientation, it's likely your partner isn't used to being really *seen* or openly looked at with desire. Unfortunately, it's not necessarily the norm for women to be in control of their own sexuality (yet), and many people find it quite exciting to be gazed at in an overtly sensual manner. As a result, that simple action can really turn up the heat and kick things up a notch!

Just remember – with great power comes great responsibility. So, be wise and use this skill carefully like you would any other effective device in your potent toolbox of sexiness.

Now that you have your smile and direct gaze down pat, let's talk about your light-hearted approach to life and its challenges.

Each day you're faced with choices. When someone pulls out in front of you in traffic, you can curse and be nasty, or you can chill out and let it go. If you spill your drink at the expensive coffee shop, you can get all flustered and embarrassed, or you can smile, crack a joke, and make light of the situation.

Which choices are easier or seem to come naturally?

Which choices do you think I'm going to recommend?

Here's another situation where it helps to think about which reactions are appealing to you. What attitude would you want to see in someone else? Aren't you always more attracted to people who manage to laugh things off and who rarely get flustered? Well – it doesn't take a rocket scientist to know that more people will be attracted to *you* if you show those same qualities.

This doesn't mean you need to behave as though nothing ever bothers you. Sometimes life sucks. You know it, and I know it. There are legitimate reasons to be upset, and I'm not suggesting you ignore them. What I'm saying is: put it all in perspective, and know which stuff you should react strongly to and which stuff you should just let pass you by.

***Here's a tip:** It's ok to let most stuff just pass you by.

Look at it this way: shit happens. It will *always* happen – usually when you least expect or want it to. Whether it's a spilled drink, the waitress messes up your order, or *you* make a mistake – how you react is the key.

At the end of the day, most of the shit that happens doesn't really matter in the grand scheme of things, so why spend the energy being wrapped around the axle over it?

Build a bridge, and get over that shit.

When you build that bridge and react with a light-hearted approach, people will notice. They will find you interesting, appealing, and want to get to know you better. That leads to more quality connections, which in turn can lead to more quality sex! That's not just great, that's WOW!

The third core characteristic of being juicy is having a persistently positive and self-confident demeanor.

That's a mouthful, isn't it?

Some women think it's both difficult to say AND to accomplish. After all, you really can't be positive and self-confident *all* the time, can you?

Sure you can!

The point here *isn't* to be some unrealistic, Pollyanna-like person who never has a bad day. That would not only be impractical, but it would likely have people wondering if you're from Stepford.

Instead, the point *is* to be positive and self-confident *at your core*. About yourself. You know – that beautiful, interesting, quirky, wonderful person that is the *only* you that exists on this planet?

This one is a bit more of a challenge to achieve, I'll admit. But I'm going to let you in on a little secret. There is a sure-fired way to develop self-confidence that's simpler than you think. The trick is...

...are you ready for it? Here goes:

Just accept your awesomeness.

---Don't worry – you can take a moment to let that sink in.

If you're like many women, as soon as you read that you possibly laughed, and your mind may have conjured up all sorts of reasons why you believe you *aren't* awesome.

Because women (more so than men) are taught to be demure and not brag about themselves, it's likely you had a thought that goes something like this: *"Oh, I know I'm awesome, but I can't act like it, because I don't want people to think I'm trying to be better than them."*

Or perhaps it was more along the lines of, *"Well – I would be totally awesome, but I'm not good at math/I need to lose weight/insert other perceived flaw here."*

Stop minimizing yourself.

Stop it. Right now.

It doesn't *matter* if you suck at math. Who *cares* if you need to lose weight?

I guarantee the **only** person who worries intensely about your flaws is you. Just shift all that energy from focusing on what you *think* is wrong with you to what you *know* is right with you, and you'll experience an immediate increase in your juiciness.

You've likely overcome some pretty big challenges in your life, and I bet you have talents/skills other people don't. Heck, if you know the first thing about algebra, you're already leaps and bounds ahead of me! Staying focused on the skills and talents you *do* have will increase your confidence.

It all boils down to this: confidence is a ridiculously sexy quality. If you're a confident woman, you exude the impression that *you are enough*. When you are enough, you approach the world from a place of wholeness, and attract partners who are healthier – both mentally and physically.

Needless to say, that definitely leads to improved intimacy, and will go a long way towards taking your sex life from great...to wow!

✳✳✳✳✳✳✳

Valuable Tips & Resources:

1. Want to learn how to "build a bridge and get over" shit? Richard Carlson wrote a phenomenal book I highly recommend, called *Don't Sweat the Small Stuff and It's All Small Stuff: Simple Ways To Keep The Little Things From Taking Over Your Life.* You can find a whole series of these helpful books at www. http://dontsweat.com. When you learn how to avoid sweating the small stuff, you'll be amazed at how much energy you free up. That's all energy you can spend on being juicier!

2. Flirt with the whole world! This doesn't mean you should try to sleep with or seduce everyone. This *does* mean to smile at children when they smile at you, find things to laugh about every day, and nurture your own inner child every chance you can. Buy some pajamas that appeal to your playful nature (I'm a fan of Tinkerbell

jammies). If there's music playing in the grocery store and you feel like dancing or singing along, *do it!* Don't worry about what people might think of you – they're probably envious that you're unabashedly enjoying yourself.

3. Check out these 25 Killer Actions to Boost Your Self-Confidence: http://zenhabits.net/25-killer-actions-to-boost-your-self-confidence/

4. If you like charts and visual aids (I know I do), check out these diagrams of 10 Simple Steps to be more interesting: http://www.forbes.com/sites/jessicahagy/2011/11/30/how-to-be-interesting/

5. Always ask other people about themselves, but also make sure you have a couple of good stories of your own up your sleeve or in your pocket/handbag (and be interesting when you tell them). Want to learn how to be a good storyteller? http://www.bakadesuyo.com/2013/03/interview-ucla-film-school-professor-howard-suber-explains-storyteller/

2. Love Yourself
(yes - it's what you think it is!)

Masturbation.

Flicking the kitten.

Clicking your own mouse.

Whatever you want to call it (there are hundreds, if not thousands, of euphemisms for self-gratification), suffice it to say, the concept makes a lot of people uncomfortable. Perhaps it even makes **you** uncomfortable?

Good - Keep reading!

Hopefully, by the time you're done with this book, you'll not only have shed that discomfort, but you will have increased your comfort level with reading about it/talking about it/***doing*** it.

Just so you know – you're not alone in your discomfort. Lots of people feel awkward talking about masturbation. I come from a liberal environment where I was raised to be very sexually open-minded, but even in that atmosphere, what people choose to do with themselves behind closed doors was only alluded to briefly, if at all, in discussions about sexuality.

In our Western culture, it's not difficult to understand why this subject is so taboo. After all, we're the only nation on the planet suffering from the Puritanical Movement. Those uptight, conservative people with the weird hats and big buckles – they ruined a lot of things for the rest of us, and masturbation is just one of them.

Even in our "enlightened" society, we don't talk about self-gratification in polite company, and stores that sell sex toys are often hidden from general view in shopping centers, with blacked out windows and large signs indicating the minimum age requirement to enter. Some religions claim masturbation is dangerous to the spirit, and some even admonish their followers that it is a sin against God.

Even so, masturbation is something much more acceptable for men to engage in, and is often highlighted in mainstream movies, usually with a comedic focus. Whether it's the hilarious end "product" in *Something About Mary*, or watching Steve Carell spend quality time with himself in *The 40 Year Old Virgin*, the message often seems to be along the lines of, "Hey – look over there – that guy's playing with his penis – isn't that funny?"

Meanwhile, female masturbation scenes in mainstream media are rare, though lately we've seen increasingly more examples. As recently as 2013, Aubrey Plaza starred in *The To-Do List*, where her character masturbated on screen.

Interestingly, when interviewed on the Conan late night show, Ms. Plaza stated she *actually* masturbated for the scene; an admission that earned her many kudos from women and girls all over America.

Thankfully, we do seem to be entering a slightly more free-thinking era of human sexuality where female masturbation is not only less denigrated, but even encouraged and celebrated. In fact, there has been a surge in businesses whose aim is to not only support women who want to increase the passion in their life, but to provide them with the toys and various accessories helpful in such pursuits.

Which is a lovely way to segue into the "nuts and bolts" of this topic – exactly *how* do we masturbate? And *why*?

I mean, if you're in a relationship with someone else, aren't *they* responsible for your orgasms? Why should you spend time making yourself feel good if you have a partner who can do it?

These are all great questions, and I'm going to address them, but let's clear something up first:

WHO Is Responsible For YOUR Orgasm: I bet you can guess what I'm going to say here, right? The only one responsible for your orgasm is you. Not your partner. Not the mail carrier. Not even your vibrator.

Which doesn't mean your partner/mail carrier/vibrator can't play a very important part in helping you climax, by the way.

Ultimately however, it's up to you, and *only you*, to make sure you achieve orgasm.

Some women don't seem to understand this concept, so I'm going to spend a bit of time on it. For those of you who totally get this and are on the same page, feel free to skip to the next section; you won't hurt my feelings.

For everyone else, ***make sure you read this next part carefully:***

Back in 2004, a girlfriend of mine and I were out having coffee and talking about life (relationships), the universe (men), and everything (relationships with men). Just when the conversation was going really well and I felt we were on the verge of solving all the world's problems, she said something that totally blew my mind.

Brace yourself, because I'm going to share it with you here.

She said, "*I'm so upset – my boyfriend has never given me an orgasm.*"

Can you believe it??

I sure couldn't! I was speechless, and even had to have her repeat herself to make sure I heard her correctly the first time. It turned out, I *did* hear her correctly – she was actually complaining that her boyfriend hadn't ever "given" her an orgasm.

Now, let's think about that for a second, shall we? What's so important about that statement?

More importantly, think about whether or not you have ever made a similar comment. Or, perhaps you've never said it outright, but maybe you've thought it? Have you ever felt "gypped" because your partner didn't "give" you an orgasm? And just what the heck is wrong with that sentence anyway?

I'll tell you, just like I told my friend, precisely what's wrong with it.

That entire approach *removes* your power and places responsibility for your orgasm squarely on someone else. Someone who is not you – and who bears no resemblance to you, other than the fact that they are probably a biped and most likely human (though if they aren't, that's ok, too).

In the case of my poor misguided girlfriend, she was placing the responsibility for her orgasm on her boyfriend. A boyfriend who was physically, sexually, emotionally, and in all other ways – *different* from her. The poor guy! Not only was that unfair to him, it clearly wasn't working for her, either.

But wait, it gets worse.

After I pointed out that an orgasm isn't like a Christmas present – you don't wrap it in shiny paper tied up with a bow and hand it to someone – I asked her if she had ever told him ***how*** to give her an orgasm. Can you guess what her answer was?

That's right – she had *never* bothered to give the poor guy any instructions at all. In fact, she told me that he should "just know" how to please her and take her to states of bliss heretofore never experienced (or something like that).

I almost choked on my overpriced coffee!

I'm sure there are many women who simply assume their partner should just magically know how to please them – and that is *sooo* not fair to either person. Whether your partner is a man or a woman (or anything else), you absolutely have to assume they have no idea how to please you, and then take it upon yourself to share that important information and guidance freely.

For more on this, read Chapter 4.

Meanwhile, returning to that conversation with my girlfriend, I decided to take a step backwards in the process, and ask her how she brings herself to orgasm when she masturbates (yes, I *do* ask the personal questions). I was totally unprepared for her response:

"Oh, no – I could *never* do that – it's yucky!"

Seriously?

Are you fucking kidding me?!?

It turns out, she wasn't kidding.

She refused to masturbate (her parents had taught her it was "bad" and "dirty"), and she had never brought herself to orgasm, yet here she was complaining that her poor boyfriend didn't "give" her orgasms, even though she had no clue how to give herself one, and had never once given her boyfriend even a hint of guidance in the matter.

OK people, this is the sexual equivalent of setting sail on a ship and expecting the captain to take you to China, even though he/she has never sailed to China, or on that particular ship, and you refuse to provide a user manual, a map, or even give a direction in which to aim. There can be no positive outcome here, folks.

The good news is, you can avoid a similar fate!

Which brings us nicely to the first of our two questions.

So – HOW do you masturbate?

Essentially, any way that is pleasurable to you while being safe, comfortable, and empowered is the *best* way to masturbate.

The first thing to focus on is the amount of time you have available. Do you have plenty of time for a long session, or do you need a "quickie"?

Certainly, if you're new to masturbating, taking your time is definitely the way to go. For some women, spending quality time with themselves requires a bed. A locked door, comfy linens, soft lights, sexy music, and an assortment of toys (or not, as you prefer) – can all go a long way towards setting a lovely scene for a successful venture in self pleasure.

Once you're cozy and relaxed, take the time to explore your body and find out what feels good. Touch yourself everywhere – learn the topography of your beautiful self. And trust me – you *are* beautiful. It doesn't matter what size you are, or whether your thighs jiggle, or how many scars you have.

Your body is good, beautiful, and strong – exactly as it is - right now in this moment.

Take as much time as you need – touching yourself, figuring out what feels good, and what doesn't. If you like visual images, there are plenty to be found on the Internet – having your laptop close by may help.

***Great Advice:** If you've never looked at your genitals in a mirror, now is the perfect time! After all, how can you guide someone else around if you don't know the geography yourself? Many women have been brought up with mixed messages about their bodies in general and about their genitals specifically, and some have even been raised with damaging stereotypes.

Please know - your body is **not** "dirty" or "bad" or any other negative words you may have been taught.

When you start touching yourself, be gentle, and watch yourself in a mirror if you can. The combination of watching while touching yourself is empowering and you might find yourself pleasantly surprised at how it makes you feel. Also, make sure you know the anatomy of your genitals. Did you know you have both inner and outer labia? Now – this isn't an anatomy guide, but you get the idea.

***For more details on your unique and beautiful self, I've included some helpful resources in the section at the end of this chapter.

If you're particularly adventurous or simply ready for something more than just your hand, dildos are great for internal stimulation, while vibrators help speed things along and provide express, powerful stimulation directly to the clitoris.

Initially, you may just focus on clitoral stimulation, which is fine. You can start with your fingers, and touch the area around your clitoris – working your way up to direct stimulation. Once you're ready, you can use a small vibrator and just go at your own pace.

Try different speeds and pressure, but remember - your clitoris has *at least* 8,000 sensory nerve endings – that's a lot! In comparison, the male penis only has about 4,000.

Furthermore, the sensations from your clitoris can spread through your pelvic area by affecting 15,000 other nerve endings.

Just like dynamite – even though your clitoris is quite small, it packs a really powerful punch!

Pretty cool, right?

In addition to your clitoris, you also have a wonderful area inside you called the "g-spot." I highly suggest you get to know this area quite well, as stimulating it can produce some seriously amazing feelings. Fair warning – some women are capable of producing more than a bit of wetness when they are stimulated, so this is a perfect time to have some towels easily accessible. In fact, I recommend you place them on the bed underneath you before you start masturbating – it can help make cleanup much easier.

And, just like the differences in skin color, gender, and preferences about pizza (I love tons of pepperoni and you might not), some women don't enjoy having their g-spot stimulated.

Just remember: don't stress yourself about it. There's no "requirement" here to do anything other than feel good. So, if you decide you don't like it, don't do it. If you decide you *do* like it, do it a lot. If you just aren't sure, keep playing around until you *are* sure.

Of course, the bed isn't the only place to masturbate – many women find a bath or shower to be a wonderful place to spend quality alone time. Whether you're in a bathtub, hot tub, or shower, a direct stream of water over your vulva and clitoris can feel simply amazing. In fact, one of those hand held shower attachments from the local hardware store might just become your new best friend. You can also try altering the force and the warmth of the water, but be careful and don't make it too hot - remember all those sensitive nerve endings!

***Important:** avoid spraying water directly into your vagina – that can do damage and possibly affect your delicate pH balance.

Once you've gotten the hang of making yourself feel really good, you may find there are times when giving yourself a "quickie" is helpful – I like to think of this more along the lines of "maintenance" orgasms. They're kind of like an oil change – get in, get it done, and get on with the day.

Just make sure you still take the occasional long date with yourself to keep exploring what feels good!

Now then - *why* would you want to masturbate?

Well, why the heck not??

Seriously – masturbation is the safest sex there is, and it's an amazing way to make yourself feel good. This creates a domino effect, because when you know how to make yourself feel good, you'll feel empowered, and that will be reflected in how you engage the world and people around you.

It is also the best way to get to know yourself, your body, and what feels good to you. This can only benefit your overall sex life, as you'll be able to share this information with your partner, and *that* will lead to better sex!

Did you know? Orgasms are great for stress release and increased focus. In fact, as recently as 2013, Rutgers researchers showed that orgasm activates the whole brain, which helps keep it sharp. Needless to say, it's a lot more enjoyable than doing crossword puzzles or Sudoku!

Another great reason to masturbate is to increase your orgasmic potential. Essentially, the more you touch yourself, the more orgasmically responsive you become. It's a fact that women who pleasure themselves when they are alone are much *more* likely to experience climax when they have intercourse with a partner.

In a nutshell, masturbating and learning to pleasure yourself is the surest way to take your partnered sexual experiences from great...to wow!

✳✳✳✳✳✳✳

Valuable Tips & Resources:

1. Start by learning your way around the lush landscape of your vulva and vagina: http://www.ourbodiesourselves.org/health-info/self-exam-vulva-vagina/

2. If you're interested in buying your own fun toys but want privacy, consider ordering online from www.pureromance.com. Founded *by* a woman and with a mission to *empower* women, they're an organization that supports women's sexual

health and independence, so you can feel good about supporting their business.

3.   If you have a couple of girlfriends with whom you feel comfortable, consider having a passion party. This is a great way to shop for fun toys in the comfort of your own home, while having adult beverages and a great time. At the end of the night, you may have a new toy and you will have supported another woman's business. It's a win-win!

4.   If you like erotica, you can spend hours scouring the Internet for something suitable while trying to avoid pop-ups and malware. Alternatively, you can start with a list of sites that has already been compiled for your reading and viewing pleasure (literally): http://www.yourtango.com/20085340/best-free-online-erotica#.VE6B4uf6jEU

5.   Pleasing yourself isn't just about your vagina – the rest of you is a luscious, sexually interesting human being who deserves the very best attention. Try seducing yourself, and spend some time with the rest of your body. Amy Levine has a great article you may benefit from (don't worry – it's free): http://www.igniteyourpleasure.com/

3. Stay Creative
(keep things spicy!)

Boredom is death.

Variety is the spice of life.

Have you ever said, or heard someone else say these phrases?

I'm here to tell you - they are both true, and absolutely important to remember when applied to your sex life.

Whether you are currently flying solo, or have been with the same person for years, keeping your sex life fun, creative, and interesting is essential. Let's face it – you are a sexual being, and your sexuality is an important part of your fabulous self.

You are far too extraordinary to have a humdrum, boring sex life!

If you're in a long-term relationship, having a boring sex life can be dangerous to the relationship as a whole. When sex is boring, it begins to feel like a chore. I don't know about you, but I hate chores! When confronted with a chore I don't want to do (like have boring sex) I can think of a hundred other things I would rather do.

Unfortunately, this approach can create distance between you and your partner. Then, it's like a row of dominos – the more distance between you, the less connected you are sexually, thus the more rote your encounters become - and the cycle continues.

To avoid that outcome, consider it a priority to keep your intimacy interesting, exciting, and varied. Yes, it takes intention, effort and energy, but it's worth it.

In addition to the emotional and personal benefits, regular (and exciting) sex has an amazing array of physical benefits, including increased endorphins, more calories burned (one of my personal favorites), and reduced stress levels.

If that's not reason enough to keep things creative, I don't know what is!

***Disclaimer:** I am NOT saying you need to have sex while wearing black vinyl & swinging from a trapeze in order to spice things up. Not that there's anything wrong with it if that's what you want to do, but there are tons of ways to keep things interesting without risking injury. Besides, black vinyl does *not* breathe, and those swings can be darned uncomfortable. But I digress…

First up: Change the scenery.

Don't get me wrong; I'm sure you adore your bed. It's probably comfy, and with fluffy pillows and high thread count sheets, it can be one of the best places to get frisky. However, if that's the only place you ever have sex, things can get a bit stale, placing you squarely in a sexual rut.

Take time to create enough privacy to try other rooms of the house. This may mean getting a babysitter, kicking the roommates out for the night, or locking pets in another room for a while.

Even your otherwise ordinary sofa can be a wonderful change of venue, and it's very design makes some positions easier than the bed (think doggie style, etc.). Pretending you're a teenager by having a "make out session" can be loads of fun – see how far you and your partner can go before removing any clothes.

Also, it may be a bit cliché, but don't discount the old "fluffy rug on the floor with a roaring fire" scenario. Curling up with your honey in front of a cozy fire can be quite romantic.

***Creative Tip:** If you live in a home without a fireplace, you can play a loop video of a fire on your TV or even your laptop. Add some candles and the right music in the background, and you have the makings of a fun evening!

***Advanced Maneuver:** Have your favorite erotica movie playing on the TV and pick a scene or a couple of positions to duplicate.

Remember in the last chapter when I suggested you try masturbating in water? Well - having sex with a partner in water can also be an intimate, sensual experience. Don't worry if you don't have an idyllic, romantic waterfall nearby, your shower will do just fine. The space may be tight, but a $12 curved curtain rod for your bathtub will give you extra space to move about.

If you're feeling a bit self conscious, simply turn off the overhead lights and light some candles. Not only does the water help keep things moving nicely, but you can clean up right after you get dirty!

Next: Be more playful & have fun!

Above all, sex *should* be fun. Otherwise, what's the point?

As important as it is to have fun when you're having sex, it's almost more important to have fun when you're *not* having sex.

That's right – when was the last time you played with your partner in a non-sexual way?

The first frisky thing to do when you're with your playmate is flirt. It's such a simple thing, really, but if you've been with the same person for years, it's one thing that may have fallen off your radar.

Remember what it was like in the beginning of your relationship when you flirted all the time? Think back to the time when just the touch of their hand made you thrill with excitement. Remember how fun it was to add sexual innuendo to your conversation, because you couldn't wait to have some sexy time with them. That was hot, right? Well - the next time you're out in public with your sweetie, no matter what you're doing, flirt with them, and bring back some of that heat!

If you're flying solo, it can be easy to put yourself in a passive position and hope someone else will take the initiative. That's not going to guarantee sparks will ever fly, though. Avoid being a wallflower and waiting for people to flirt with you. Allow yourself to be empowered enough to initiate the flirting!

Most importantly, flirt *without being attached to the outcome*. This is key - just flirt and be fun with the only intent being to convey interest – don't have your expectations set on whether or not the other person flirts back.

I'm fond of saying expectation is the mother of disaster. When you flirt without expectation of the outcome, you'll find yourself lighter, more carefree, and *much* more empowered. Then, if something does happen, it's just icing on the cake!

Another way to get the juices flowing with your dearest is to engage in a friendly game of competition. If your interests lean more towards the cerebral, how about a nice game of chess (or scrabble, etc.)? To make it even more interesting, take your game to the local park and play there. Doing something playful, different, and outside your usual surroundings will definitely help keep things creative.

If you and your partner are into more physical pursuits, challenge them to something fun and physical like basketball. Make sure to keep things light hearted and fun, but also work hard enough to break a sweat and have some full body contact.

Once you have those endorphins flowing, there's no telling how well you can heat things up.

***Creative Tip:** to kick the spice level up a notch, increase the stakes, and have the loser give the winner a sexy body rub. That will really get things humming along in the right direction!

Finally: Think outside the box!

The best way to keep your sex life varied, creative, and fun is to think outside the box.

Believe it or not, this is a bit more difficult than it sounds. If you're like most women, you may have a gazillion things you need to focus on, and trying to come up with creative ideas for sexy fun can seem like just one more thing to add to the list.
Usually, it falls somewhere towards the bottom – after laundry, cooking, cleaning, errands, etc.

Lucky for you, thinking outside the box only takes a small amount of thought, a dash of creativity, and a focus on fun. Once you get the hang of it, you'll find it even easier to come up with your own creative ideas, but here are some great tips to get you started!

First, think about all the games you had fun playing when you were a kid. For instance, scavenger hunts come to mind – who didn't love those? There's something exciting about solving clues and not knowing what's at the end of the trail.

For outside-the-box fun, send your partner on a sexy scavenger hunt. You can write up some flirty clues, and they can find you waiting at the end of the trail – as dressed or undressed as you please!

***Important Note About Lingerie:** Please know that you do NOT have to wear some corset/garter belt/high-heeled contraption that feels like it was invented by the Marquis de Sade just to be sexy! Your lingerie should be something you *actually* feel sexy in, and not just something the marketing companies tell you that you *should* feel sexy in.

If you feel sexy in an attractive apron and nothing else, great! If you have a cute pair of boy shorts and an oversized t-shirt that make you feel fabulous, wear them! Obviously, try for something more than just your old sweats, but stick to what you feel comfortable in and what makes you feel good.

Speaking of oversized t-shirts, if you have a lover who is really into watching televised sports, take a note from my playbook and buy an oversized jersey from their favorite team. On game day, wear the jersey - and not much more. Spend the commercial breaks acting as their personal cheerleader, and see what happens.

If you and your honey lean towards the traditional and enjoy dinner and a movie, try switching it up. With your laptop and some basic picnic supplies, you can find a secluded spot and create your own drive-in movie. If it's too cold outside, just move the living room furniture out of the way, toss a blanket (or Twister game) on the floor, and have yourselves a romantic carpet picnic.

Whatever you do, just remember – keeping life fun, flirty, and interesting *outside* the bedroom can result in more sexy fun *inside* the bedroom, and take your overall intimacy level from great…to wow!

✶✶✶✶✶✶

Valuable Tips & Resources:

1. For those of you without a fireplace, check out this handy YouTube video of a cozy, crackling fire: http://youtu.be/BLmwmX-mni8

2. Invest in some bathtub soap "crayons" or make your own. You can buy them from Amazon for about $10 or so, and if you're super crafty (I'm not) you can make your own with unique shapes and custom colors. Then, when your partner isn't around, use the crayons to write a sexy message on the shower wall. Something like, "meet me here at a certain time for some clean/dirty fun" – you get the idea.

3. If you haven't used sexy coupons with your partner, now's the time! If you're creative and have the time, you can make your own. You can also Google them – there are tons of sites out there that offer different options and make it easy to print out some fun, sexy love coupons. This is just one of those sites: http://archive.lovingyou.com/content/passion/passionplay-content.php?ID=eroticcoupons

4. Thanks to Women's Health, here are eight MORE ways to make sex creative: http://www.womenshealthmag.com/sex-and-relationships/make-sex-more-fun

5. If you want boards games geared more towards adults, here's a great list of a few to get you started: http://www.more.com/sexy-board-games-couples

4. Communicate Clearly
(say what??)

Talking.

Sexting each other.

Playing show and tell.

There are tons of ways to communicate about sex – do you have a preference?

Or, like many women, do you find yourself slightly uncomfortable sharing your wants/needs/desires with your lover?

I'm fond of saying, "If you don't ask, you don't get." Needless to say, this *most definitely* applies to your sexual desires.

Remember that girlfriend of mine I told you about in Chapter 2? The poor girl wasn't in touch with her own sexuality, which pretty much guaranteed an inability to communicate her needs.

Even if she *had* been in touch with her own desires, the fact that she never clearly communicated those desires to her boyfriend resulted in significantly underwhelming sexual experiences for her and, I'm guessing, for him as well.

Unfortunately, communication challenges aren't only the domain of the young and inexperienced. If you find yourself a bit tongue tied or apprehensive about having such intimate conversations, don't worry – you're not alone!

Engaging in clear, direct conversations about sexual preferences can be intimidating and challenging – even for the most mature, well-spoken woman. If you want to take your sex life from great to wow, you definitely need to overcome these challenges.

To conquer any insecurity you may have when it comes to talking about your needs and those of your lover, take a moment to re-apply what you learned in Chapter 1 - *just accept your awesomeness*.

Look at it this way: Anyone you choose as a sexual partner has also chosen you – most likely, because you're simply fabulous! Odds are, they want to make sure your mutual sexual experiences are as excellent as they can be.

So - how can you more easily engage in the necessary *verbal* intercourse with a goal of improving your *sexual* intercourse?

First of all, timing is key:

In those gloriously intimate moments after sex, take the opportunity to talk about your preferences (and those of your sweetheart) while you're still enjoying that post-coital afterglow. This is an excellent time to have this discussion because everything is still fresh in your mind. Also, for many people, shyness is less of a challenge after an orgasm.

Seize the opportunity to snuggle up, ask a couple of "passion questions," and start some sexy dialogue. Phrasing your questions properly can be enormously helpful as well. Using the words "I'm curious" before your question lets your partner know you're truly interested in their answer.

The best questions to ask are often the most basic. Starting with *"What did you like?"* is an excellent way to receive a positive response. Meanwhile, although the flip side of that coin is also important, asking your lover about what they *didn't* enjoy doesn't necessarily have to be a negative turn in the discussion.

***Important:** For afterglow conversations, be sure to listen attentively, and keep the focus *positive* and informative.

Building on those inquiries, you can move on to asking what they might like more of, or even what they might like to try next time.

"But what if they say they like/want something I think is just gross?"

Yep – I'm not gonna sugar coat it – that may very well happen. One person's turn *on* can be another person's turn *off*, but you'll never know unless you ask!

If that does happen, above all, remain tactful. It may be challenging for your partner to admit they have a certain proclivity, and it won't help matters if you respond with an outburst of, *"EWWW – That's just GROSS!"*

After all, you wouldn't want them to say something like that to you, would you?

The best thing to do in this situation is to politely say something like, *"That's interesting. I'll admit – it doesn't appeal to me; is there another way I can help you get this need met or something else we can do that works for both of us?"*

Responding in this way lets your lover know you're listening to them without judgment and that you are truly interested in finding ways to satisfy them that work for you both. That in turn will help ensure they continue to feel comfortable opening up to you about their intimate preferences.

Hopefully, your honey will be 100% into everything you tell them about your needs & desires, but the reality is that they may not be. That's totally fine – as long as you're both loving and supportive of each other during the discussion.

It's always helpful to preface your desires with a disclaimer that lets your partner know you aren't going to insist that they like what you like, and that you won't hold it against them if they have a different preference.

Whatever your sweetie shares with you, make sure you keep an open mind and listen intently. *You may be pleasantly surprised at what you learn!*

Think about other ways to communicate:

Beyond talking with each other, there are additional ways to communicate that may work well for you.

One creative option is to use writing as your method of interaction. You can each write a brief note or letter to the other, detailing what you would like to share. Taking time to do this in a place of privacy is helpful. And, since you're not face to face with them, you may feel empowered to give more detailed descriptions than you would otherwise.

If you like the written word, taking a field trip together to a library or bookstore can be both fun AND enlightening. Hit up the sex manual section (sometimes found in self-help) and each of you pick a book (or a couple) to peruse.

Remember - keep a sense of playfulness about you; sex is supposed to be fun, remember?

One way to make this field trip effective is to carry some colored sticky notes and a pen with you. Take a half hour or so, and spend some time placing the notes on the pages of the book(s) you've chosen, and you can even include some writing or other sexy ideas on the sticky notes.

When the time is up, switch books. Take this opportunity to check out each other's notes and develop a few sexy ideas about what you both might enjoy the next time you get together.

Not only can this be an enjoyable and informative experience, it can also be a creative type of foreplay.

***Fair Warning:** spending time reading and thinking about sex, pleasing your partner, and being pleased might get one or both of you aroused. You may want to make sure your schedule is clear afterward so you can take advantage of all those sexy ideas you stir up!

Finally, make sure you show...AND tell!

Sometimes, one of the best ways to get a message across is to show someone what you mean.

When you're indulging yourselves in each other's bodies, take advantage of the moment. Praise the things your lover does that make you feel good. Make sure you take the time to guide their hands, mouth, or other body parts to the places on your body where you crave attention.

It can be quite helpful (*and sexy!*) to talk to your partner during sex – and tell them what you like *while* you're showing them. A perfect example of this is to take their hand, place it where you like to be touched, and at the same time tell them, "I really love it when you touch me here/like this" or "It gets me so hot when you do this____" – and then guide them through whatever it is that gets you hot.

Don't just focus on *your* needs though – make sure you're giving at least as good as you get (and better, if possible). Compliment your partner on how they look, taste, and feel. Tell them how much you love making them feel good, and follow up your words with actions. Odds are, they'll mirror those actions back to you, further increasing your mutual satisfaction levels.

Remember - everything you and your lover share about your preferences is simply raw material to improve your next sexual experience together, and take it from great…to wow!

Valuable Tips & Resources:

1. Talking dirty during sex can be hot – but it can also be awkward. Here's a great article to help you talk dirty without feeling like an idiot! http://www.bustle.com/articles/29263-how-to-talk-dirty-with-your-partner-without-feeling-like-an-anti-feminist-idiot

2. Are you looking for a book you can use to show your partner positions you might like to try? This book has 365 to choose from! http://books.google.com/books/about/365_Sex_Positions.html?id=XlHPQpyB5jUC

3. On your field trip to the bookstore, take along some fun & flirty sticky notes for all your sexy comments and tips! http://www.post-it.com/wps/portal/3M/en_US/PostItNA/Home/Products/~/Post-it-Super-Sticky-Notes-3-in-x-3-in-Heart-Shapes-Pink-2-Pads-Pack?N=4327+3294646034&rt=rud

4. This is an overall great site with lots of excellent tips, including how to talk about sex: http://www.goodinbed.com/blogs/sex_doctors/2011/02/how-to-talk-about-sex/

5. Searching for the right word when you're talking about sex can be a bit challenging. Thankfully, there's a helpful site that will greatly add to your current vocabulary: http://www.sex-lexis.com

5. Keep Practicing
(practice makes ~~perfect~~ **progress!**)

Ideally, this would be the shortest chapter in the book. There shouldn't be anything but the heading and a blank page. After all, it's self-explanatory, right?

Not exactly.

Did you know? Your sensuality and sexuality are just like muscles – they tend to atrophy when not regularly used.

Thankfully, the opposite is also true - the more frequently you have, or even just *think* about having sex, the more you tend to want it. The day-to-day challenge is that it is far easier to focus on your shopping list, calendar of activities, projects due at work, family issues…well, you get the idea.

As a result, it's no surprise that it takes conscious effort to practice thinking about sex (and not just thinking about how much you *aren't* having).

It's also important to practice actually *having* sex- both with yourself and with a partner (if you have one). Even the experts agree, as evidenced by this excerpt from a 2012 article in Psychology Today:

> "Practice masturbating a few times a week to start and try and work your way up to masturbating or being sexual with your partner every other day. You will begin

developing an appetite for being sexual with better frequency if you are being sexual on a regular basis. You will also begin building sexual self-confidence as you learn how your body reacts and what feels good to you."

***For the entire article, I've included the link in the resource section at the end of this chapter.

Keeping your sensual muscles in shape isn't the only reason to practice sex regularly. Remember all those great tips on keeping things spicy and creative from Chapter 3? Well, following creative suggestions once or twice can be fun and certainly add spiciness to your intimacy.

But what happens when you *stop* being creative?

Without regular practice and application of a creative approach, your intimacy levels are likely to revert to where they were previously. That's fine if you're comfortable in a sexual rut, but if you were, you wouldn't be reading this book in the first place!

Beyond keeping you out of that sexual rut, there are so many other reasons to consider your sexuality an important life practice (like yoga or meditation), they can fill an entire book of their own.

Here are some key highlights:

If you want to keep fit (*and who doesn't?*), have sex regularly!

That's right - even just 30 minutes of "vigorous" sex can burn up to 100 calories. Over the course of a year, that can really add up!

I'm not great at math, but even I can calculate those results. Let's say you have a couple of sessions of moderately intense sex each week. By the end of the year, you will have burned somewhere around 6,000 extra calories. That's definitely tastier than the grapefruit diet, and a lot more enjoyable than going to the gym!

Speaking of working out, if you engage your creativity and practice different positions during all this sexy fun, you'll also make progress towards being more bendy and flexible. It's the most fun way I can think of to strengthen and tone multiple muscle groups.

Did you know? Besides working your muscles, every time you're sexually active, your body releases pheromones that help make you attractive to others. The more frequently you have sex, the more pheromones you secrete, and the more attractive you are to others!

Of course, attraction-inducing pheromones aren't the only chemicals your body releases during sex. Even being intimate only once or twice a week will allow your body to increase levels of other helpful compounds, including flu-fighting antibodies. I don't know about you, but that sounds so much more enjoyable than getting a flu shot!

For those of you who want to stay young longer but don't want to go to the extremes of plastic surgery or becoming a vampire, you'll be happy to know that having sex releases natural steroids and anti-ageing hormones into your body.

Among the numerous hormones let loose as a result of sex are estrogen, which helps smooth out wrinkles (*yay!*), and DHEA, which boosts your immune system. This means you'll be less prone to being sick AND you'll look and feel younger, longer. I'd definitely say that's a win-win!

All of these examples are proof that when you practice improving and enhancing your sexuality and intimate creativity on a regular basis, many areas of your life will go from great...to WOW!

✳✳✳✳✳✳✳

Valuable Tips & Resources:

1. As promised, here's that great article from Psychology Today: http://www.psychologytoday.com/blog/save-your-sex-life/201206/women-only-guide-coming-out-your-sexual-shell

2. Need more reasons to have regular sex? http://www.mirror.co.uk/lifestyle/health/21-reasons-you-should-sex-2043200

3. For the science nerd in all of us, here's an interesting site that talks about the hormones of sex – from Adrenaline to Vasopressin: http://www.youramazingbrain.org/lovesex/sciencelove.htm

4. Here's a great workout specifically designed to help you have **better** sex: http://www.shape.com/blogs/fit-list-jay-cardiello/best-sex-workout-youll-ever-have

5. ...and here are 10 great sex positions that double as **great** exercise! http://www.fitnessmagazine.com/mind-body/sex/sex-positions-that-double-as-exercise/

www.ingramcontent.com/pod-product-compliance
Lightning Source LLC
Chambersburg PA
CBHW071330310526
45789CB00017B/2180